I CAN KEEP CALM I'M TURNING 50

Birthday Gift Notebook
(7 x 10 Inches)

Name:

Phone:

E-Mail:

www.InspirationalWares.com

Goals:

- [ ]
- [ ]
- [ ]
- [ ]
- [ ]
- [ ]
- [ ]
- [ ]
- [ ]
- [ ]

Accomplishments:

○
○
○
○
○
○
○
○
○
○

Habit Tracker	1	2	3	4	5	6	7	8	9	10

Appointments & Special Dates:

For more amazing journals and adult coloring books from Penelope Pewter, visit:

Amazon.com
CreateSpace.com
RWSquaredMedia.Wordpress.com

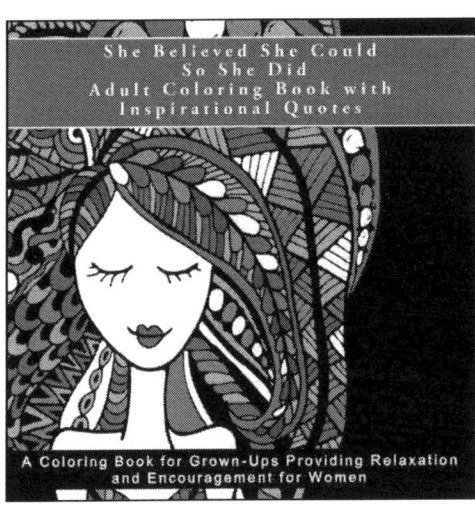

She Believed She Could
So She Did Adult Coloring Book
with Inspirational Quotes

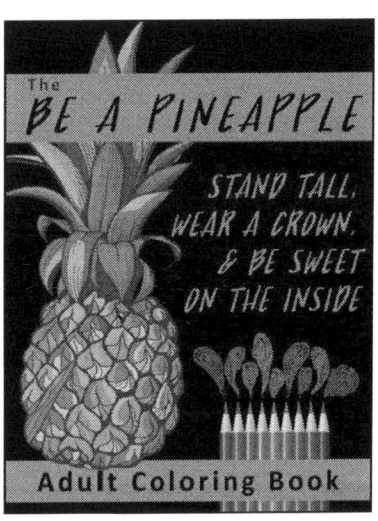

The Be A Pineapple Adult
Coloring Book

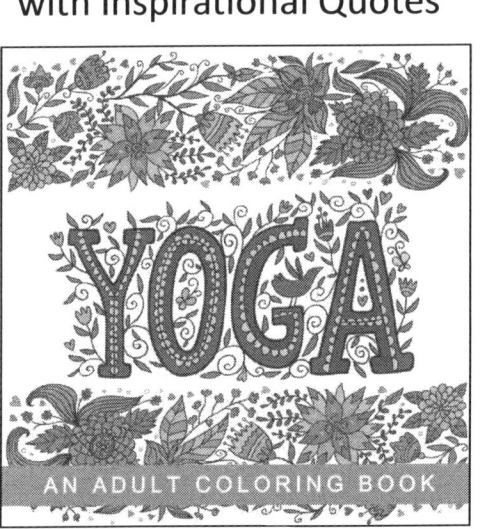

YOGA
An Adult Coloring Book

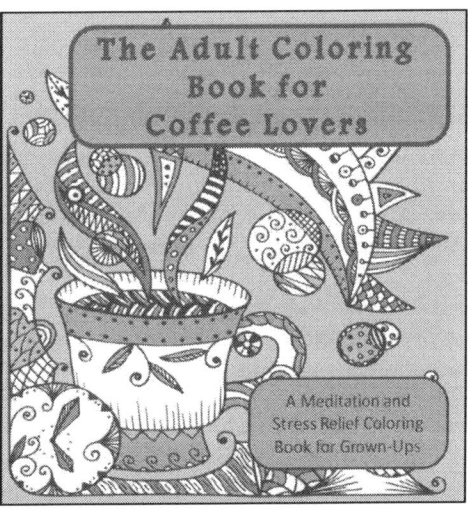

The Adult Coloring Book for
Coffee Lovers

InspirationalWares.com

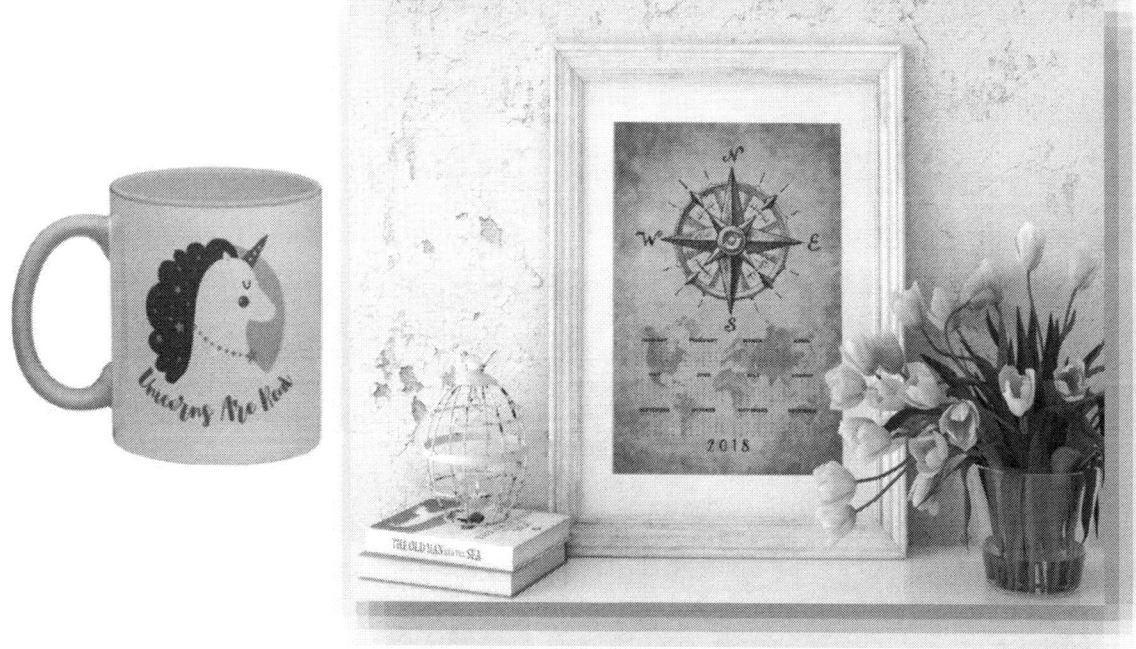

Funny & inspirational calendars, posters, coffee mugs and more!

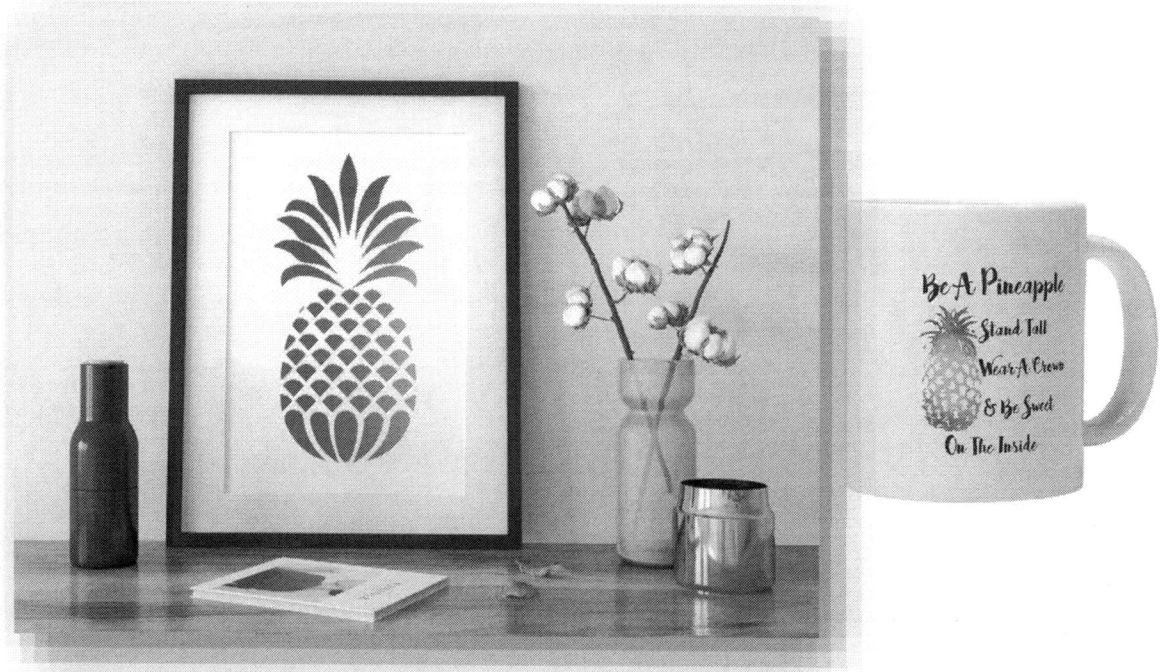

https://InspirationalWares.com

Printed in Great Britain
by Amazon